Contents

What Is The 17-Day Diet?

The 17 Day Diet was created by Dr. Mike and promises quick weight loss—10 to 15 pounds over the first 17 days—through a restrictive first phase that eliminates sugar, grain-based foods, fruit, and most dairy foods. The diet claims to rev up your metabolism and encourage your body to burn fat.

It's suggested to help you lose weight rapidly and build healthy eating habits. The key to this diet is constantly changing foods and calorie intake, which is claimed to boost your metabolism.

The 17 Day Diet is divided into four cycles: Accelerate, Activate, Achieve and Arrive. The first three cycles last 17 days each, while the Arrive cycle is meant to be followed for life.

As you move through the cycles, the diet introduces new strategies and food options.

It's worth noting that the diet does not tell you how many calories to eat during each cycle. However, it progressively increases your calorie intake by introducing more calorie-rich options with each cycle.

Proponents of the diet tout its fast results (especially during the first 17 days), and many have found that it's easy to implement and follow. However, as with any diet, it's tricky to get sustained results, and people who have followed the 17-Day Diet say it's difficult to follow long-term.

How Does The Diet Work

If you have food allergies or intolerances, following the 17-Day Diet should be relatively simple—you'll just need to eliminate the foods you can't have. For those with nut or dairy allergies, it's easy, since those foods are mostly not included in the diet blueprint. It's also easy to follow the diet if you follow a gluten-free diet since it mentions when you can have foods such as gluten-free bread and gluten-free pasta.

The program also includes "transitional day fasts," which are supposed to "coax your body into additional fat-burning between cycles." These fasts are optional, according to Dr. Moreno. If you choose to do the transitional day fasts, you'll consume smoothies in three liquid meals on your fasting days. The smoothies contain almond milk, yogurt, whey powder, powdered fiber, plus fruit.

There are four phases, or "cycles," on the 17-Day Diet, the first three of which are 17 days long. Here's a breakdown of each cycle.

Cycle 1: Accelerate

The first cycle of the 17 Day Diet is the Accelerate cycle.

It claims to help you lose 10–12 pounds (4.5–5.4 kg) over the first 17 days by (1):

- Increasing your protein intake.
- Improving digestive health.
- Reducing sugar, sweets and refined carbs.
- Clearing your body of possible toxins that affect your metabolism.

During this phase, you're allowed to eat unlimited protein and vegetable options from the specified Accelerate foods list. Most carb-rich foods are banned during this cycle.

However, fruits are an exception — though you're not allowed to eat any fruit after 2 p.m. The book claims that it is harder to burn carbs later in the day, as you're less active.

Other guidelines to follow include:

- Purchase skinless poultry or remove the skin.

- Avoid alcohol and sugar to improve digestion.

- Consume two probiotic foods daily to promote digestive health.

- Eat slowly and chew thoroughly until you feel full.

• Drink eight 8-ounce (240-ml) glasses of water each day.

• Exercise at least 17 minutes per day.

Cycle 2: Activate

The second cycle of the 17 Day Diet is the Activate cycle.

During this cycle, you alternate between lower- and higher-calorie days.

On lower-calorie days, you simply eat as you would during the Accelerate cycle. On higher-calorie days, you can add two servings of naturally higher-starch carbs, such as legumes, grains, tubers and root vegetables.

To follow this cycle, spend one day on the Accelerate plan, the next day on the Activate plan. Continue to alternate between these two versions over the next 17 days.

This second cycle is based on the idea of alternate-day fasting. However, it takes a modified approach, as its lower-calorie days are higher in calories than on a traditional alternate-day fasting diet.

In addition, the Activate cycle adds plenty of new food options.

This cycle is claimed to help reset your metabolism, but evidence to support this is lacking.

Many rules form the Accelerate cycle still apply, such as not to eat carbs after 2 p.m. This means that you must eat your carb options with breakfast and lunch during this second cycle.

Cycle 3: Achieve

The third cycle of the 17 Day Diet is the Achieve cycle.

This cycle aims to establish healthy eating habits with steady, manageable weight loss. Alternate-day fasting is no longer required and the diet is similar to the Activate days of the second cycle.

You are now allowed to eat a wider variety of carb sources, such as breads, pastas, high-fiber cereals and virtually any fresh fruit or vegetable.

Since you're eating more food than in previous cycles, it's recommended to increase aerobic exercise from the minimum 17 minutes to 45–60 minutes per day.

It's worth noting that it's still not permissible to eat carbs after 2 p.m. during this cycle.

Cycle 4: Arrive

The last cycle of the 17 Day Diet is the Arrive cycle.

Unlike other cycles — that all last 17 days — this cycle is meant to be followed for life.

For this phase, you may choose any meal plan from either of the three previous stages — Accelerate, Activate, Achieve — and follow them from Monday breakfast to Friday lunch.

From Friday dinner through Sunday dinner you can enjoy your favorite foods in moderation. However, you're advised not to eat more than one to three of your favorite meals over the weekend.

In addition, you can drink one to two alcoholic beverages daily over the weekend.

It's recommended to get in at least an hour of intense exercise on Saturday and Sunday since you consume more calories on the weekends.

During this cycle, it's still suggested to not eat carbs after 2 p.m.

Will 17 Day Diet help you lose weight?

Likely. It'll be hard not to lose weight with the balanced diet and regular exercise this diet prescribes, consuming fewer calories than your body burns is a surefire way to lose weight .

For instance, during the Accelerate cycle, the 17 Day Diet limits your choices to lean proteins, non-starchy vegetables and probiotic foods — which are low in calories.

During the Activate phase, it implements a modified take on alternate-day fasting, which has been found to be effective for fat loss, as people find it easy to follow.

Still, though the diet can aid weight loss, it makes various weight loss claims that are unsupported by evidence, such as that the change in food groups and calorie intake can "confuse" and boost your metabolism.

It also recommends avoiding carbs after 2 p.m., claiming that carbs eaten later in the day are harder for your body to burn, as you burn less energy in the evening. However, there are no high-quality studies that support this claim.

How much should you exercise on 17 Day Diet?

Exercise is a key component of the 17 Day Diet. During the first and second cycles, you'll spend 17 minutes each day doing light exercise, like walking. During the third cycle, you'll do 40 to 60 minutes of aerobic exercise "most" days of the week. In the final cycle, you'll exercise for an hour on weekends and keep up your regular regimen on weekdays.

Is 17 Day Diet a heart-healthy diet?

Unclear, but its meals are low in fat, cholesterol and sugar, which should decrease your risk of heart disease and high blood pressure. Regular exercise will also strengthen your heart and lower your chances of high cholesterol, high blood pressure and clogged arteries (atherosclerosis).

Can 17 Day Diet prevent or control diabetes?

No studies have looked at the 17 Day Diet for diabetes, but balanced eating and regular exercise can help prevent and control the condition.

Prevention: Being overweight is one of the biggest risk factors for Type 2 diabetes. If this diet helps you lose weight and keep it off, you might tilt the diabetes odds in your favor.

Control: A diabetes diet should be low in sugar and refined carbohydrates to keep blood sugar levels in check – this regimen limits both. And because there are no rigid meal plans or prepackaged foods, you can ensure that what you're eating doesn't go against your doctor's advice.

Certain fruits like pineapple, watermelon and bananas are high in sugar, and they don't promote fat loss. Too much sugar from any source can load your body into converting more of what you eat into stored body fat.

Fruit shouldn't be avoided entirely, it's just important that you make the right choices when selecting fruit for your snack. Most berries are low in sugar, as well as fruits like cantaloupe.

Just be moderate in how much you eat—two servings a day, only.

Research indicates that probiotics boost the immune system and help rid the body of bad bacteria.

Probiotic foods have also been shown to help burn body fat. One of the best probiotics available for a snack is low-fat yogurt.

If you don’t like yogurt, try sugar-free fruit-flavored yogurt or cultured milk, such as low-fat acidophilus milk (it tastes just like regular low-fat milk). Most health food stores sell capsules containing probiotics; just make sure you follow the manufacturer's guide if you are going to take these supplements.

Is This Diet Right for Vegetarians?

The 17 Day Diet is appropriate for vegetarians with plenty of option. If you're a "lacto-ovo-vegetarian", you can limit your protein to dairy products and eggs. That means you'll obtain your protein from probiotics like yogurt, eggs, and beans and legumes (depending on which cycle you are on). "Semi-vegetarians", who avoid red meat but eat fish or chicken, can easily follow the diet. "Vegans" avoid all animal proteins. If you're a vegan, you can still follow the diet. Simply use vegan meat substitutes at meals for protein and use a probiotic supplement in place of yogurt.

What Kind of Snacks Should I Eat?

The 17 Day Diet recommends adding fruit and probiotics to your plan.

Certain fruits like pineapple, watermelon and bananas are high in sugar, and they don't promote fat loss. Too much sugar from any source can load your body into converting more of what you eat into stored body fat.

Fruit shouldn't be avoided entirely, it's just important that you make the right choices when selecting fruit for your snack. Most berries are low in sugar, as well as fruits like cantaloupe. Just be moderate in how much you eat—two servings a day, only.

Research indicates that probiotics boost the immune system and help rid the body of bad bacteria.

Probiotic foods have also been shown to help burn body fat. One of the best probiotics available for a snack is low-fat yogurt.

If you don't like yogurt, try sugar-free fruit-flavored yogurt or cultured milk, such as low-fat acidophilus milk (it tastes just like regular low-fat milk). Most health food stores sell capsules containing probiotics; just make sure you follow the manufacturer's guide if you are going to take these supplements.

What To Eat

The eating plan on the 17-Day Diet reduces the intake of carbohydrates by eliminating all refined carbohydrates and sugars. The diet does allow for some whole grains and prioritizes low-carb vegetables, lean protein, and healthy fats. The 17-Day Diet works in cycles, with different foods allowed during different cycles.

The program includes three meals per day plus snacks. The goal is to keep people who are following the diet from getting hungry. From the first cycle, you can eat as much as you want of specific proteins and the so-called "cleansing" (e.g., non-starchy) vegetables.

The diet blueprint includes suggested meal plans for all days, although you can mix and match those plans to suit your own tastes. You also can elect to do fast days in between the cycles (in which you'll consume smoothies) to supposedly jump-start your weight loss.

To follow the 17-Day Diet, it's helpful (although not required) to purchase Dr. Moreno's book, which includes meal plans and recipes along with the diet blueprint. Still, most meal templates are simple. For example, a typical breakfast in Cycle 2 includes one cup of lean granola with 6 ounces of no-sugar-added fruit-flavored yogurt, while a typical dinner would feature garlic shrimp, steamed green beans, and a large tossed salad dressed with 1 tablespoon olive oil.

Food to Eat

- Fish and low-fat poultry (Cycle 1)
- Shellfish and higher-fat poultry (Cycle 2)

- Poultry, bacon, and sausage (Cycle 3)
- Red meat (Cycles 2 and 3)
- Eggs (all cycles)
- Non-starchy vegetables (all cycles)
- Starchy vegetables (Cycles 2 and 3)
- Legumes (Cycles 2 and 3)
- Whole grains (Cycles 2 and 3)
- Probiotics (e.g., yogurt, kefir, sauerkraut) (all cycles)
- Low-sugar fruit (e.g., apples, berries, pears, citrus) (all cycles)
- High-sugar fruit (e.g., bananas, mango, pineapple) (Cycle 3)

Food To Avoid

- Milk, ice cream, and most other dairy products (all cycles)
- Foods with added sugar
- White bread (and other highly processed bread products)
- Candy
- Wheat flour-based pasta
- Dried fruit
- Flavored coffee drinks
- Juice

The 17-Day Diet focuses on eliminating certain carbohydrates from your meals. Therefore, you'll tend to eat more protein than you might normally while eliminating entire groups of carb-based foods.

Protein

There are plenty of protein options on the 17-Day Diet, even starting in the diet's more restrictive first cycle. From day one, you can enjoy fish (including salmon, sole, flounder, catfish, tilapia, and canned light tuna in water). You also can have chicken and turkey breast, lean ground turkey, and eggs in limited quantities. In the second cycle, you can add shellfish, lean red meat, lamb, and veal. In the third cycle, you can have fatty types of poultry plus turkey bacon, turkey sausage, and Canadian bacon.

Vegetables

When it comes to vegetables, the 17-Day Diet breaks them down into two categories: starchy and non-starchy. Non-starchy vegetables, which Dr. Moreno calls "cleansing vegetables," are allowed in unlimited quantities. They include cauliflower, cabbage, broccoli, Brussels sprouts, asparagus, celery, green beans, greens, mushrooms, onions, and tomatoes. Starchy vegetables are allowed beginning in Cycle 2. They include corn, potatoes, pumpkin, sweet potato, and winter squash.

Fruit

Fruits are also divided into two categories: low-sugar fruit and high-sugar fruit. Two servings per day of low-sugar fruit are allowed from the first cycle, while high-sugar fruit isn't allowed until the third cycle. This diet categorizes low-sugar fruits as apples, berries, grapefruit, oranges, peaches, pears, plums, prunes, and red grapes. High-sugar fruit includes apricots, bananas, cherries, figs, kiwi, mango, papaya, pineapple, tangelo, and tangerines.

Grains

The diet bans grains and other "natural starches" in Cycle 1, but then allows them (limited in types and quantities) in Cycles 2 and 3. In Cycle 2, you can add amaranth, barley, brown rice, couscous, cream of wheat, grits, long-grain rice, millet, oat bran, old-fashioned oatmeal, and quinoa. In Cycle 3, your grain-based options expand dramatically, with whole-grain and gluten-free bread, high-fiber cereals, plus various kinds of pasta (whole wheat, gluten-free, vegetable-based, and high-fiber).

Dairy

Dairy products are allowed in moderation on the 17-Day Diet. In Cycles 1 and 2, people following the program are encouraged to have two servings per day of probiotic foods, which include yogurt, kefir, and acidophilus milk, along with Breakstone Live-Active cottage cheese (cottage cheese with active cultures).

In Phase 3, they can add small amounts of certain cheeses (Brie, camembert, fontina, low-fat cheddar, Edam, feta, goat, Limburger, and part-skim mozzarella). They also can enjoy low-fat cottage cheese, low-fat milk, and low-fat ricotta cheese.

Fats

When it comes to fats, Dr. Moreno encourages people following his program to consume 1 to 2 tablespoons of "friendly fats" (olive oil and flaxseed oil) from the first day. Once they get to Cycle 3, they also can have a small amount of avocado, canola oil, walnut oil, mayonnaise, nuts or seeds, reduced-calorie margarine, and salad dressing per day.

Benefits and Drawbacks

Benefits

- Diet relies heavily on healthy vegetables and lean protein
- Easily accommodates dietary restrictions
- Followers are likely to lose weight, especially at first

Drawbacks

• May not provide enough fiber, particularly in beginning

• Difficult to follow long-term

• Requires lots of food prep and meal planning

Though some health experts say that evidence for the 17-Day Diet is lacking, according to Dr. Moreno's website, there is some science behind it. Review the pros and cons to inform your decision about trying this diet.

Benefits

• Lots of veggies and lean protein. The 17-Day Diet's cycles include loads of healthy non-starchy vegetables and lean protein. In fact, you're allowed to have unlimited amounts of both in all phases of the diet. These should help prevent hunger in the diet's early days.

- Adaptable to dietary restrictions. If you have celiac disease, a dairy intolerance, or a nut allergy, you can easily tailor the program to meet your needs. Food choices are expansive enough that you can steer clear of allergenic items and still follow the diet.

- Weight loss is likely. You're almost certain to lose a significant amount of weight, especially in the diet's early days. That's because your calories will be pretty limited, even though you can have unlimited lean protein and non-starchy vegetables. Initial weight loss can boost motivation and may also improve energy and sleep, which can help you stay on track with your new healthy eating plan.3

Drawbacks

• Not enough fiber. Everyone needs fiber—in fact, current dietary guidelines recommend anywhere from 22–28 grams of fiber per day for adult women and 28–34 grams for adult men. If you are not careful with planning out your meals in the first cycle, you could fall shy of your fiber needs. Be sure to incorporate lots of non-starchy vegetables and two servings of high fiber fruits daily to meet your daily needs.

• Confusing to follow. The initial phase of the 17-Day Diet can be difficult to follow as it has very specific rules and food restrictions. However, the later stages appear to be more balanced. Some people may find it time-consuming to prep and cook meals, however, the recipes are fairly simple.

Health Benefits

While proponents of the 17-Day Diet claim that it will speed up the body's metabolism and lead to increased weight loss, research supports that any weight loss resulting from temporary diets is often not sustained. Even though the fourth phase of the diet is meant to be lifelong, many people may have a hard time sticking with it.

However, the eating plan does tout the benefits of cutting back on refined carbohydrates and added sugars and emphasizes lean protein and fresh vegetables, which could help people develop healthy eating habits for the long term.

Health Risks

While there are no common health risks associated with the 17-Day Diet, it does lack dietary fiber during the first cycle. Research has shown that getting enough fiber is necessary for maintaining digestive health, reducing inflammation, and preventing colon cancer.

17-Day Diet Food List

The 17-Day Diet is divided into four different cycles, which means that what you eat will vary depending on which cycle you're in. The most restrictive phase of the diet is Cycle 1, but the eating plan starts to ease up during Cycle 2. On "Cycle 2" days, you can eat everything that was allowed during Cycle 1 with the addition of higher-fat protein, whole grains, starchy vegetables, and legumes. The following shopping list includes the basics for Cycle 2 and includes foods from Cycle 1. Note that this is not a definitive shopping list, and you may find other foods that work better for you.

Cycle 1: Accelerate

- Low-carb vegetables (asparagus, zucchini, broccoli)

- Olive oil and flaxseed oil

- Lean protein (tofu, white-fleshed fish, low-fat cottage cheese)

- Low-sugar fruit (mixed berries, grapefruit, avocado)

- Probiotic foods (kefir and tempeh)

Cycle 2: Activate

- Higher-fat meats and fish (chicken, beef, salmon, shrimp)
- Whole grains (quinoa, brown rice, barley, low-fat granola, rolled oats)
- Starchy vegetables (potatoes, sweet potatoes, butternut squash)
- Legumes (chickpeas, beans, lentils)
- Fruits (apples, nectarines, pears, grapes)
- No-sugar-added yogurt (plain or with fruit added)

The 17-Day Diet: A Sample Menu

There's no strict meal plan. Instead, the 17 Day Diet lists acceptable lean proteins, nonstarchy vegetables, low-sugar fruits, natural carbohydrates and dairy that you can choose from in certain proportions. While the acceptable-foods list changes slightly during each of the diet's four cycles, in general you'll be eating things like grilled chicken, scrambled egg whites, fat-free yogurt, fresh berries, salad and steamed broccoli. Seasonings are usually fat-free or homemade. And don't worry about feeling hungry – as long as you don't overeat, there are few portion regulations on this plan.

Diet soda and coffee are allowed, but not necessarily recommended. You're instructed to drink at least eight glasses of water a day, which might be tough if you're sipping other beverages as well.

Here is a one-day sample menu for each cycle of the 17 Day Diet.

Accelerate cycle

- Breakfast: 6 ounces (170 grams) of plain, low-fat yogurt, 1 cup (150 grams) of berries and 1 cup (240 ml) of green tea.
- Lunch: Grilled chicken breast with tossed salad drizzled with 2 tablespoons (30 ml) of balsamic vinegar.
- Dinner: Grilled or baked chicken with steamed vegetables and 1 cup (240 ml) of green tea.
- Snacks: 1 fruit of your choice and 1 serving of a probiotic food of your choice.

Activate cycle

- Breakfast: 1/2 cup (230 grams) of cooked oatmeal, 4 scrambled egg whites, 1 peach and 1 cup (240 ml) of green tea.

- Lunch: Shrimp salad drizzled with 2 tablespoons (30 ml) of balsamic vinegar, 1 medium baked sweet potato and 1 cup (240 ml) of green tea.

- Dinner: Meat sirloin chops (broiled or grilled), steamed veggies and 1 cup (240 ml) of green tea.

- Snacks: 1 cup (150 grams) of blueberries and 1 cup (240 ml) of kefir.

Achieve cycle

- Breakfast: 1 slice of whole-wheat toast, 1 boiled egg, 1 cup (150 grams) of berries and 1 cup (240 ml) of green tea.

• Lunch: Tuna sandwich, 1 pear and 1 cup (240 ml) of green tea.

• Dinner: Sesame fish, steamed vegetables of your choice and 1 cup (240 ml) of green tea.

• Snacks: 1 frozen fruit bar and 6 ounces (170 grams) of yogurt.

Arrive cycle (Friday)

• Breakfast: 2 poached eggs, 1 pear and 1 cup (240 ml) of green tea.

• Lunch: Baked turkey breast, a fresh garden salad drizzled with 1 tablespoon (15 ml) of flaxseed oil, 6 ounces (170 grams) of yogurt and 1 cup (240 ml) of green tea.

• Dinner: Dinner out with friends; for example, vegetable lasagna, tossed salad with blue cheese dressing, two 5-ounce (150-ml) glasses of red wine and 1 serving of tiramisu.

• Snacks: 1 apple and 1 cup (240 ml) of acidophilus milk or 6 ounces (170 grams) of yogurt.

17-DAY DIET RECIPES

Trying 17 day-friendly recipes is a great way to explore new flavors and find new favorite dishes while looking after your health. In this part are nourishing 17-day diet recipes for you to enjoy.

Veggie Egg Cups

Prepartion time

45 minutes

Ingredients

- 1 16oz carton of egg whites plus 2 whole eggs (lightly beaten) (may use Egg Beaters)
- 1 chopped green onion
- 1 large handful cherry tomatoes, sliced (or more)
- 1/3 cup of frozen spinach, thawed
- 1 red or green bell pepper, chopped
- 1/4 cup shredded Parmesan cheese
- Salt & pepper to taste

Instructions

1. Preheat oven to 350 degrees F.

2. In a large bowl, mix all ingredients together. Pour mixture into greased muffin tins or silicone baking cups.

3. Bake for approximately 30-35 minutes or until toothpick comes out clean.

Egg Roll in a Bowl a la Judy

Prepartion time

30 minutes

Ingredients

- 1 Tablespoon sesame oil (may use Olive Oil)

- 1 pound ground chicken (may use turkey for C1, or beef or pork for C2)
- 2 bags 1-pound cole slaw mix (cabbage/carrot mix) (a total of 2 pounds)
- 2 red onions chopped
- 10 cloves fresh garlic, minced
- 1-3 teaspoons ground ginger, to taste
- red pepper flakes (optional)
- 1/4 to 1/2 cup low-sodium light soy, to taste
- salt and pepper to taste
- 1/4 cup chicken broth or water
- 2-3 green onion stalks finely chopped (optional for garnish)

Instructions

1. On medium heat, heat oil and brown meat in large frying pan until fully cooked.

2. Increase heat to medium high and add chopped onions and slightly brown.

3. In a small bowl, mix garlic, ginger, soy sauce and add to pan.

4. Immediately add cabbage/carrots mix and cook through until cabbage is semi-wilted, but still have a crunch to them.

5. Add chicken broth or water as needed if mixture is too dry.

6. Salt and pepper to taste.

7. Garnish with chopped green onion and serve.

Waffle Omelettes

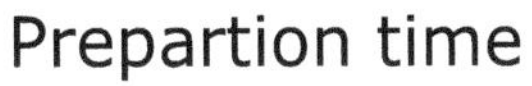

Prepartion time

20 minutes

Ingredients

- 2 Eggs
- 4 Egg Whites
- 1/4 cup onion, finely chopped
- 1/4 cup Bell Pepper (any color), finely chopped
- 1/4 cup Spinach, chopped
- 1/4 cup tomato, chopped (or use canned tomatoes)
- Salt and Pepper, to taste

- Cheese for topping
- Salsa for topping (optional)
- Olive Oil Cooking Spray

Instructions

1. Preheat waffle iron.
2. In a small bowl, whisk together your eggs and egg whites.
3. Spray the hot waffle iron with an Olive Oil spray.
4. Sprinkle an even layer of vegetables on each waffle section and cook for about one minute.
5. Next, pour the whisked egg mixture over the vegetables, season with salt and pepper.

6. Close the waffle iron and cook until the eggs are thoroughly cooked.

7. Cooking time will vary depending on how hot your waffle iron cooks.

Asparagus and Eggs

Prepartion time

12 minutes

Ingredients

- 5-6 stalks Asparagus
- 1 teaspoon olive oil

- 2 eggs
- ¼ cup Parmesan cheese (optional)
- Salt and Pepper, to taste
- Your favorite herbs for topping (optional)

Instructions

1. Heat olive oil in pan over medium heat.
2. Cut off ends of asparagus and add to skillet along with salt and pepper to taste.
3. Toss the asparagus in the skillet to fully coat in oil and seasonings and cook until tender, 4-5 minutes.
4. When the asparagus is finished cooking, spread asparagus out and add a bit more oil (if

necessary) and crack eggs in the center and season eggs with salt and pepper.

5. Sprinkle cheese over asparagus and eggs. Cover and let cook until egg whites are firm and yolk is done to desired consistency.

Blueberries and Cream Green Smoothie

Prepartion time

10 minutes

Ingredients

- 1 Cup Spinach
- 1 Cup Plain Low-fat yogurt

- 1 ½ Cups Blueberries (fresh or frozen)

Instructions

1. Blend spinach and yogurt first.

2. Add blueberries and blend again.

3. Depending on thickness of smoothie, you made add a bit of water to thin it out, if desired or use Kefir instead of yogurt. Depending on the ripeness of your fruit, you may add Stevia to sweeten the smoothie.

Chicken Cabbage & Broccoli Stir Fry

Prepartion time

30 minutes

Ingredients

- 2 Tablespoons Olive Oil, divided
- 1 pound ground chicken
- 1 small onion, thinly sliced
- 1 red bell pepper, thinly sliced
- 1 cup matchstick carrots
- 2 Cups Broccoli Florets, cooked al dente
- 3 cloves fresh garlic, minced
- 1-2 teaspoons ground ginger or 1 Tablespoon fresh ginger
- red pepper flakes (optional)
- 1-pound bag coleslaw mix (cabbage/carrot mix)

- ¼ cup light soy sauce, or more if desired
- ¼ cup water, or more if needed
- salt and pepper to taste
- 2 green onions finely chopped, reserve some for garnish

Instructions

1. On medium heat, heat oil and brown ground chicken in large frying pan until fully cooked.
2. Remove from pan, cover and set aside.
3. In the same pan, heat remaining olive oil and sauté onions until they become tender.
4. Add sliced bell pepper and matchstick carrots and sauté for about two minutes.

5. Add in al dente broccoli florets and stir to combine.

6. In a small bowl, mix garlic, ginger, soy sauce and water and add to pan.

7. Next, add the cooked chicken back to the pan and stir to combine.

8. Immediately add cabbage/carrots mix and cook through until cabbage is semi-wilted, but still have a crunch to them.

9. Add green onions and warm through (reserve a few to garnish)

10. Add water if mixture is dry.

11. Salt and pepper to taste.

12. Garnish with remaining chopped green onion and serve.

Middle Eastern Turkey and Carrot Stew

Prepartion time

1 hour

Ingredients

- 1 pound lean ground turkey
- 2 small onions, diced
- 1/2 bulb garlic, minced
- 3 carrots, halved and sliced
- 1/2 teaspoon nutmeg
- 1/2 teaspoon allspice

- 1 teaspoon cinnamon
- 1 teaspoon salt
- 1 teaspoon pepper
- 1 teaspoon coriander
- 1 small can tomato juice (V8) *or* 1 small can tomato sauce (Torey's edit)
- 14 oz can diced tomatoes
- 1/2 cup water
- Steamed Broccoli or brown/basmati rice for serving (optional)

Instructions

1. In a large pan over medium-high heat, add turkey and brown.

2. Next, add vegetables to turkey mixture and sauté until onions are tender.

3. Add spices to mixture to toast, about 1 minute.

4. Add tomatoes, tomato juice and water and simmer until carrots are tender, about 30 to 40 minutes.

Chicken Enchilada Soup (Slow Cooker)

Prepartion time

8 hours 20 minutes

Ingredients

- 1 1/2 pounds boneless skinless chicken breasts
- 1 medium onion, diced
- 1 bell pepper, thinly sliced
- 1 jalapeño, de-seeded and diced
- 1 Serrano chili, de-seeded and minced
- 2 cloves garlic, minced
- 1 15-oz. can diced tomatoes
- 2 cups chicken stock (or broth)
- 1 Tablespoon chili powder
- 1 Tablespoon cumin
- 1 teaspoon dried oregano
- 1/2 teaspoon paprika

- Salt and pepper, to taste
- 2 Tablespoons fresh cilantro, chopped (optional)
- Low-Fat Sour Cream (optional)

Instructions

1. Add the chicken to the bottom of the slow cooker.

2. Add the onion, bell pepper, jalapeño, Serrano chili, and garlic on top of the chicken.

3. Next, pour the diced tomatoes and chicken stock over the top.

4. Sprinkle with the spices and seasonings over the top.

5. Cover and cook on low heat for 8 hours.

6. Use a fork to shred the chicken before serving.

7. Garnish with cilantro and a dollop of low-fat sour cream.

Unstuffed Cabbage Casserole

Prepartion time

30 minutes

Ingredients

- 1 pound Ground Lean Turkey (or chicken)
- 2 Tablespoons Olive Oil
- 1 Small Onion, chopped
- 1 teaspoon Garlic Powder
- 1/2 teaspoon Onion Powder
- 1/2 teaspoon Dried Thyme
- 1/4 teaspoon Ground Pepper
- 1/2 teaspoon Salt
- 15 ounce Can Diced Tomatoes
- 1 Small Head Small Green Cabbage - chopped
- ½ Cup Water
- 1 Cup Low-fat Mozzarella Cheese
- Salt/Pepper To Taste

- 1 Cup Riced Cauliflower, cooked

Instructions

1. In large pot or pan, over medium high heat, brown turkey with olive oil and onions.

2. Reduce heat to medium; add garlic powder, onion powder, thyme, salt and pepper and stir until well combined.

3. Add diced tomatoes and water to mixture and bring to a boil.

4. Add cabbage, cover and reduce heat to medium low. Cook 7 to 10 minutes.

5. While mixture is cooking, prepare the cooked riced cauliflower. In a food processor or with a

grater, rice your cauliflower into rice-sized pieces. Use enough cauliflower to yield 1 cup riced.

6. In an un-oiled pan over medium heat, cook the cauliflower until all moisture is gone, about 6-8 minutes. Set aside.

7. When your meat mixture is finished cooking, cooked riced cauliflower to pot and let flavors marry for a minute or two.

8. Top with cheese and cover 1-2 minutes to melt.

9. Remove from heat and serve.

Chicken Lombardy

Prepartion time

30 minutes

Ingredients

- 2 Large Boneless, Skinless Chicken Breasts, cut in half length-wise
- 2 Tablespoons Olive Oil, divided
- Small Carton of Sliced Mushrooms
- Small Onion, diced
- 1 teaspoon Italian Seasoning
- 2 garlic cloves, minced
- ½ Cup Chicken Broth
- 2 oz cream cheese
- 1 Cup Shredded Mozzarella Cheese

- ½ Cup Parmesan Cheese
- Salt and Pepper to taste

Instructions

1. Preheat oven to 450 degrees F.

2. Season chicken with salt and pepper.

3. In a large skillet, heat 1 Tablespoon Olive Oil on medium high heat. Brown chicken breasts on each side for 3 to 4 minutes.

4. Place browned chicken into a baking dish. Set aside.

5. Add 1 Tablespoon Olive Oil to skillet and add mushrooms, onions and Italian Seasoning and sauté until mushrooms start to become tender and onions translucent, about 5 to 7 minutes.

6. Season mushroom mixture with salt and pepper and add garlic cloves and sauté for anther 30 seconds.

7. Next, add chicken broth and cream cheese to skillet and mix well to combine lifting any brown bits from the bottom of the skillet.

8. Once cream cheese has melted and sauce is thickened up a bit, pour the sauce mixture over the chicken.

9. Top chicken and sauce with mozzarella cheese, followed by Parmesan cheese.

10. Bake for about 10 to 15 minutes, or until chicken is cooked through. Baking time will depend on thickness of chicken.

11. Once cooked through, place under the broiler to allow the cheese to brown.

12. Serve immediately.

Chicken Tikka Masala

Prepartion time

45 minutes

Ingredients

For the Garam Masala Spice Blend:

- 1 ½ teaspoons ground cumin
- 1 ½ teaspoons ground coriander
- 1 teaspoon black pepper
- 3/4 teaspoon ground cardamom
- 3/4 teaspoon ground cinnamon

- 1/3 teaspoon ground nutmeg

For the ginger, onion and garlic mixture:

1. 1 1/2-inch fresh ginger, peeled and grated OR 3 teaspoons ground ginger
2. 4 cloves garlic, finely minced
3. 1/2 large yellow onion, finely diced

For the Remaining Recipe:

- 4 boneless skinless chicken breasts, diced into 1-inch cubes
- Garam Masala spice blend, divided (see above)
- Salt
- 2 Tablespoons olive oil, divided

- 1 Tablespoon tomato paste
- 1 1/2 teaspoon ground paprika
- 1/4 teaspoon cayenne pepper, or to taste
- 1 28 oz can crushed tomatoes
- 1/2 cup plain Greek yogurt
- 1 Tablespoon fresh lemon juice

Instructions

1. Mix all Garam Masala spices together and set aside.

2. Combine ginger, garlic and onion in a small bowl and set aside.

3. In a large bowl, add chicken, 1 ½ teaspoons of the Garam Masala spice blend and 1 teaspoon salt and thoroughly coat chicken.

4. Heat 1 Tablespoon olive oil in large pan on medium-high heat. Add chicken and cook on all sides until thoroughly cooked, about 6 to 8 minutes.

5. Transfer chicken to plate and cover with foil. Set aside.

6. In the same pan, add remaining 1 Tablespoon olive oil on medium-high heat. Add ginger, garlic and onion mixture to pan and cook until onions are soft.

7. Next, add tomato paste, remaining Garam Masala spice blend, paprika and cayenne pepper

to onion mixture and cook until well combined. Add crushed tomatoes and season with salt.

8. Bring tomato mixture to a boil, reduce heat and simmer for a few minutes uncovered. If mixture is too thin, simmer until it reaches a desired consistency. Add water if it's too thick.

9. Add chicken to tomato mixture and heat through, about 1 minute. Remove from heat and add in Greek yogurt and lemon juice.

Bang Bang Chicken Kebabs

Prepartion time

45 minutes

Ingredients

- 4 boneless skinless chicken breasts cut into 1-inch chunks
- 1 red bell pepper cut into 1-inch chunks
- 1 medium yellow onion cut into 1-inch chunks
- Wood or metal skewers
- Olive oil, salt, black pepper
- 1/4 cup Greek yogurt
- 1/4 cup Thai Sweet Chili Sauce
- 5-6 or more drops of Sriracha Hot Sauce, to taste

Instructions

1. Soak your wood skewers in water for about 30 minutes so that they don't burn on the grill.

2. Season the chicken and veggies with salt and pepper to taste, then drizzle with about 1 Tablespoon olive oil. Skewer the chicken.

3. Thread the red peppers and onions on separate skewers.

4. Pre-heat your grill or grill pan to medium high heat then add the chicken and veggies to the pan. Rotate the meat and veggies every few minutes to ensure food is cooked evenly.

5. When the vegetables are tender, remove them from the grill.

6. While the chicken is finishing cooking, combine Greek yogurt with Thai Sweet Chili

Sauce and Sriracha Hot Sauce in a small bowl and whisk until sauce is smooth.

7. During the last few minutes of the chicken cooking, use a brush to spread the hot sauce over the chicken.

8. Rotate the chicken and brush the other side with the sauce.

9. Remove from grill and allow the chicken to rest for a few minutes before serving.

Faux Chocolate Pudding

Prepartion time

5 minutes

Ingredients

- 3/4 cup Plain Greek Yogurt
- 1 package Truvia (or other approved sweetener)
- 1 Tablespoon unsweetened cocoa

Instructions

1. Place all ingredients in a small bowl and stir to thoroughly combine.

2. Top with your favorite low-sugar berries.

Low-Fat Low-Carb Mini Cheesecakes

Prepartion time

40 minutes

Ingredients

- 6 oz. low fat cream cheese, room temperature
- 1/2 cup part skim ricotta cheese, room temperature
- 1 egg and 1 egg yolk (beaten),
- 2 teaspoons sweetener (Stevia) (use 2 tablespoons if you prefer a sweeter cake)
- 1 teaspoon vanilla extract

Instructions

1. Preheat oven to 350 degrees.

2. Spray regular size muffin pan with non-stick spray (use cupcake liners instead if you prefer).

3. Add all ingredients to a large mixing bowl.

4. Beat with an electric mixer until mixture is smooth.

5. Divide batter evenly into 6 muffin cups.

6. Bake for 28 to 30 minutes, or until a toothpick inserted in the center of a cake comes out clean.

7. Let cool on rack.

8. Gently remove mini cheesecakes from pan.

9. Use your favorite berries for a topping or eat plain!

Ann's Creamy Fruit Freeze

Prepartion time

2 hours 10 minutes

Ingredients

- 1 cup Plain Greek Yogurt
- 1 Tablespoon Sour Cream
- 1 teaspoon Pure Maple Syrup
- 1/2 cup Berries (Ann used raspberries)
- 1/2 cup Unsweetened Applesauce

Instructions

1. In a large bowl, mash berries and stir in the remaining ingredients.

2. Freeze for one hour.

3. Remove from freezer and allow to thaw just enough to stir again.

4. Return to freezer for another hour.

5. Remove, stir and serve.

17 day diet Turkey Taco Salad

Prepartion time

25 minutes

INGREDIENTS

- Brown and drain 1 lb lean ground turkey.
- Add 1 envelope of your favorite taco seasoning or add onion , garlic, chili powder, cumin, salt and pepper to taste.
- Add 1 can diced tomatoes with liquid.
- Add 1/4 can water and stir. Cook over med heat until most of liquid is reduced.
- Meanwhile chop 1 med head of lettuce and divide on 4 plates. Dice 1 cup fresh tomatoes and one cup onion.
- Top with taco meat, tomatoes, onion, 1/4 cup grated Kraft fat free cheddar cheese, 2 tbl spoons fat free sour cream and salsa.

Instructions

1. simmer meat miixture til almost dry.

2. For cycles 2 and above add 1 can black or pinto beans to meat if desired.

Spinach-Berry Salad

Prepartion time

12 minutes

INGREDIENTS

- 1/3 cup almonds, slivered

- 4 cups baby spinach
- 3/4 cup strawberries, quartered
- 1 tablespoon balsamic vinegar
- 1 teaspoon Dijon mustard
- 1 teaspoon honey
- 3 tablespoon extra virgin olive oil
- 1 ounce soft goat cheese
- Salt and pepper to taste

Instructions

1. Place the almonds in a dry skillet or saute pan.

2. Cook over low heat, shaking the pan the entire time until the almonds are toasting. The

almonds are done when you start to smell a "nutty" scent.

3. Remove almonds from the pan to cool. (Do not cool in the skillet because they will burn from the heat that remains in the pan.)

4. Prepare the dressing by placing the vinegar, mustard, and honey in a mixing bowl. Slowly whisk in the oil.

5. Place the spinach in a large bowl.

6. Add the strawberries, almonds, and dressing.

7. Toss to coat.

8. Top with goat cheese. If desired, season with a pinch of salt and pepper.

9. Serve immediately.

Asian Chicken Salad

Prepartion time

5 minutes

INGREDIENTS

- 2 cups cooked chicken, skin removed, cut into bite-sized pieces
- 4 cups cabbage, shredded
- 1 cup mushrooms, sliced
- 1 cup carrots, grated
- 2 tablespoons cilantro, chopped
- 1 cucumber, thinly sliced
- 3 green onions, thinly sliced

- 1 mandarin orange or tangerine, divided into sections
- 1/2 cup nonfat Asian or Oriental-style salad dressing
- Black pepper

Instruction

1. In a large bowl, combine chicken, cabbage, mushrooms, carrots, cilantro, cucumber, and dressing.
2. Toss well.
3. Top with green onions and tangerine sections. Pepper to taste.

17 Day Diet, Cycle 1: Turkey Meatloaf

Prepartion time

1 hour 15 minutes

INGREDIENTS

- 1 lbs Ground Turkey, Lean
- 1 Egg, large
- 1/4 cup Scallions, chopped
- Handful of Spinach, fresh
- 2 tbsp Worcestershire Sauce
- 1 tsp Salt
- 1/2 tsp Poultry Seasoning
- 1/8 tsp Cracked Balck Pepper

- 2 tsp Garlic Salt (use garlic powder for less salt)

Instructions

1. In a large bowl, mix all ingredients together with a whisk, except the ground turkey and spinach.

2. When mixed well, add the turkey and spinach.

3. Use your hands to knead the mixture together.

4. Shape into a loaf about 1.5-2.5 inches thick.

5. Bake at 350 degrees for 1 hour or until done.

Garlic and Ranch Turkey Burger

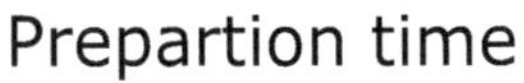

Prepartion time

30 minutes

INGREDIENTS

- 1 lb ground turkey
- 1 package ranch dressing mix
- 1 egg
- 3 gloves garlic, minced
- 1/4 cup Worcestershire sauce

Instructions

1. Preheat an outdoor grill for medium-high heat, and lightly oil the grate.

2. Knead together the turkey, ranch mix, egg, garlic, Worcestershire sauce, seasoned salt, and pepper in a bowl until evenly combined; divide into 4 equal portions and form into patties.

3. Cook on the preheated grill about 5 minutes per side for well done. An instant-read thermometer inserted into the center should read 165 degrees F (74 degrees C).

Salsa Turkey Burgers

Prepartion time

12 minutes

Ingredients

- 1 lb ground turkey (99% fat free)
- 1/3 cup seasoned bread crumbs
- 4 tbsp chunky salsa (use medium or hot for extra kick)

Instructions

1. Combine all ingredients until well mixed.
2. Add salt and pepper to taste.
3. Divide into 4 patties.
4. Spray a frying pan with cooking spray and cook over medium heat until cooked thoroughly (about 10 minutes), flipping once about half-way through.

Cucumber and Tomato Salad

Prepartion time

5 minutes

INGREDIENTS

- 1 lg. cucumber diced
- 1 med-lg. tomato diced
- 1 sm-med onion diced
- 2 cups water
- 5 tbsp. vinegar (or to taste)
- Salt (to taste)
- Black Pepper (to taste)

Instructions

1. Place diced vegetables into bowl. Add vinegar, water, salt, pepper. Mix. Refrigerate to marinate.

2. Goes great with spaghetti!

Spinach-Berry Salad

Prepartion time

12 minutes

Ingredients

- 1/3 cup almonds, slivered
- 4 cups baby spinach

- 3/4 cup strawberries, quartered
- 1 tablespoon balsamic vinegar
- 1 teaspoon Dijon mustard
- 1 teaspoon honey
- 3 tablespoon extra virgin olive oil
- 1 ounce soft goat cheese
- Salt and pepper to taste

Instructions

1. Place the almonds in a dry skillet or saute pan.

2. Cook over low heat, shaking the pan the entire time until the almonds are toasting. The

almonds are done when you start to smell a "nutty" scent.

3. Remove almonds from the pan to cool. (Do not cool in the skillet because they will burn from the heat that remains in the pan.)

4. Prepare the dressing by placing the vinegar, mustard, and honey in a mixing bowl. Slowly whisk in the oil.

5. Place the spinach in a large bowl. Add the strawberries, almonds, and dressing. Toss to coat.

6. Top with goat cheese. If desired, season with a pinch of salt and pepper.

7. Serve immediately.

P's Olive Oil & Balsamic Vinegar Dressing (2 Tbsp)

Prepartion time

10 minutes

INGREDIENTS

- balsamic vinegar
- olive oil, garlic
- salt
- pepper

Instructions

1. press the garlic and shake it all together. each serving is 1 T vinegar and 1 T oil.

Balsamic Oil & Vinegar Salad Dressing

Prepartion time

5 minutes

INGREDIENTS

- 2/3 cup Extra Virgin Olive Oil
- 1/3 cup Balsamic Vinegar
- 1 tsp minced garlic (fresh or from a jar)
- 1 tsp Cracked Pepper
- 1 packet of Splenda

Instructions

1. Mix all ingredients in an air tight container.

2. Mix or shake until thoroughly blended.

3. Shake each time you use it. Keep it in the fridge.

4. A little of this goes a long way. It coats your salad really well. Despite the high caloric and fat content, the lack of sodium (overly-abundant in most salad dressings) and the monounsaturated fat in this dressing are well worth it.

Broiled Asparagus

Prepartion time

20 minutes

INGREDIENTS

- 20 spears fresh asparagus
- 1 tablespoon olive oil
- 1/4 teaspoon salt
- 1 tablespoon black pepper

Instructions

1. Turn the broiler on.
2. Take one asparagus spear and hold at each end.
3. Bend spear until stalk breaks.
4. Take that spear and cut the rest of the asparagus at the same spot as the broken spear.

5. Put asparagus in a large bowl and pour olive oil over asparagus.

6. Toss together and put asparagus on a broiling pan.

7. Salt and pepper asparagus and put in broiler.

8. Cook for 10 minutes, shaking pan occasionally.

9. Asparagus should be light golden brown on tips and tender.

Ground Beef Cabbage Stir-Fry

Prepartion time

20 minutes

INGREDIENTS

- 1 tbsp olive oil
- 1/2 head cabbage
- 1/2 lb. ground beef, lean or ground turkey
- 1/2 green bell pepper, cut in strips
- 1/2 cup onion, chopped
- 1/2 cup sliced carrots
- 2 tbsp soy sauce
- 1/4 cup water
- 1/2 tsp pepper

Instructions

1. In large saucepan or wok, heat olive oil over med-high heat.

2. Add ground beef/turkey and cook, stirring occasionally until browned.

3. Add peppers, onions and carrots and heat over med-high heat, stirring frequently for 2-3 minutes.

4. Add cabbage, soy sauce, water and pepper.

5. Cover and reduce heat to med-low.

6. Cook about 10 minutes or until veggies are tender.

7. Serve over brown rice.

Ground Turkey & Cabbage

Prepartion time

40 minutes

INGREDIENTS

- 1 Package 99% Lean Ground Turkey (approx 1 lb)
- I Head of Cabbage
- 2 cans diced tomatoes (the new flavored kind are best)
- 3 cloves of garlic
- 1 small onion, or a couple shallots
- Salt and Pepper to taste

Instructions

1. Spray a large pot or skillet with cooking spray, sautee the garlic and onions until they are just starting to get soft, add the turkey and sautee all together until the ground turkey is just browned.

2. Chop the cabbage and add to the turkey mixture, add the two cans of diced tomatoes and stir until mixed.

3. Reduce heat and simmer for approx 30 minutes or until cabbage is cooked to the consistancy that you wish.

Stir fry green beans

Prepartion time

5 minutes

Ingredients

- 1 1/2 pounds fresh green beans, trimmed and cut into 1 inch peices
- 1 1/2 tsp sesame oil
- 1 1/2 tsp reduced sodium soy sauce
- 1 tsp sugar

Instructions

1. Heat oil over medium-high heat in a skillet or wok.
2. Add the green beans and stir fry for 3 minutes for al dente, or longer for desired crispiness.

3. Add soy sauce and stir fry 1 minute.

4. Add sugar and stir fry 30 seconds.

www.ingramcontent.com/pod-product-compliance
Ingram Content Group UK Ltd.
Pitfield, Milton Keynes, MK11 3LW, UK
UKHW022006190726
13853UKWH00004B/1765

9 798506 555056